Taking Care of Myself

# Mental Health

By Meg Gaertner



level 2 little blue readers

www.littlebluehousebooks.com



Little Blue House is distributed by North Star Editions:
sales@northstareditions.com | 888-417-0195

Produced for Little Blue House by Red Line Editorial.

Photographs ©: Shutterstock Images, cover, 4 (bottom), 7 (top), 7 (bottom), 9, 10 (top), 10 (bottom), 12–13, 15, 16–17, 18 (top), 18 (bottom), 21, 23, 24 (top right), 24 (bottom left), 24 (bottom right); iStockphoto, 4 (top), 24 (top left)

**Library of Congress Control Number: 2021916806**

**ISBN**
978-1-64619-496-4 (hardcover)
978-1-64619-523-7 (paperback)
978-1-64619-574-9 (ebook pdf)
978-1-64619-550-3 (hosted ebook)

Printed in the United States of America
Mankato, MN
012022

# About the Author

Meg Gaertner enjoys reading, writing, dancing, and being outside. She lives in Minnesota.

# Table of Contents

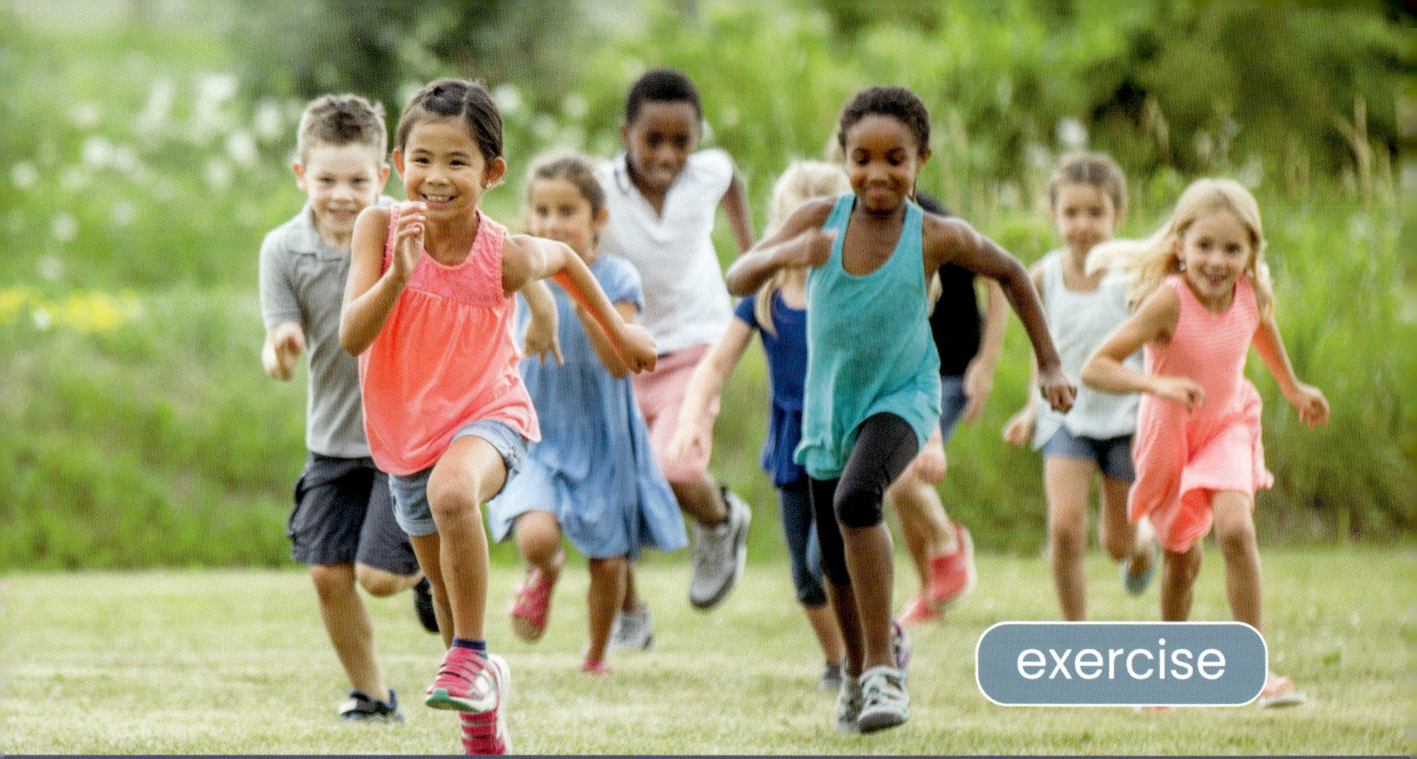
exercise

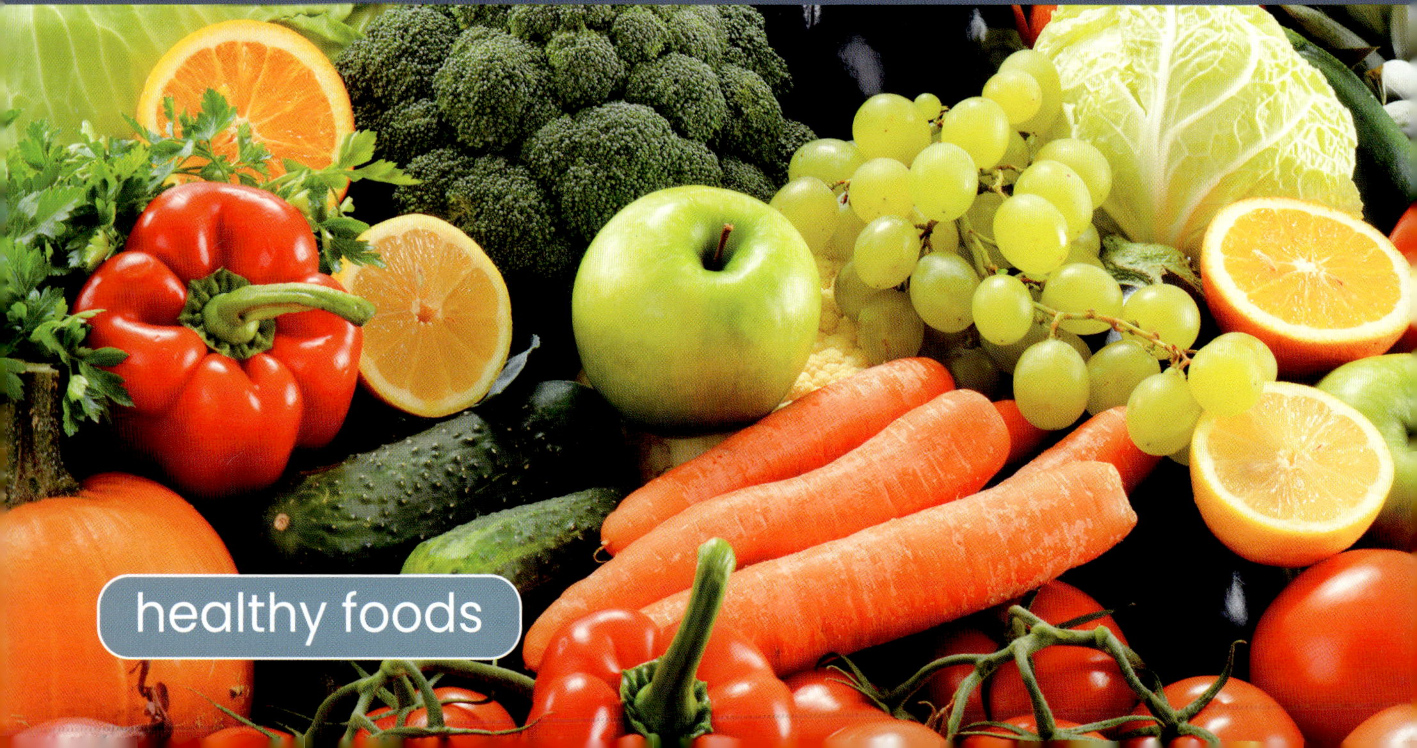
healthy foods

# Mental Health

People take care of their bodies by exercising and eating healthy foods. People take care of their minds by practicing mental health.

Mental health does not mean being happy all the time.

People become sad, mad, lonely, or worried.

Mental health means being able to handle these different feelings.

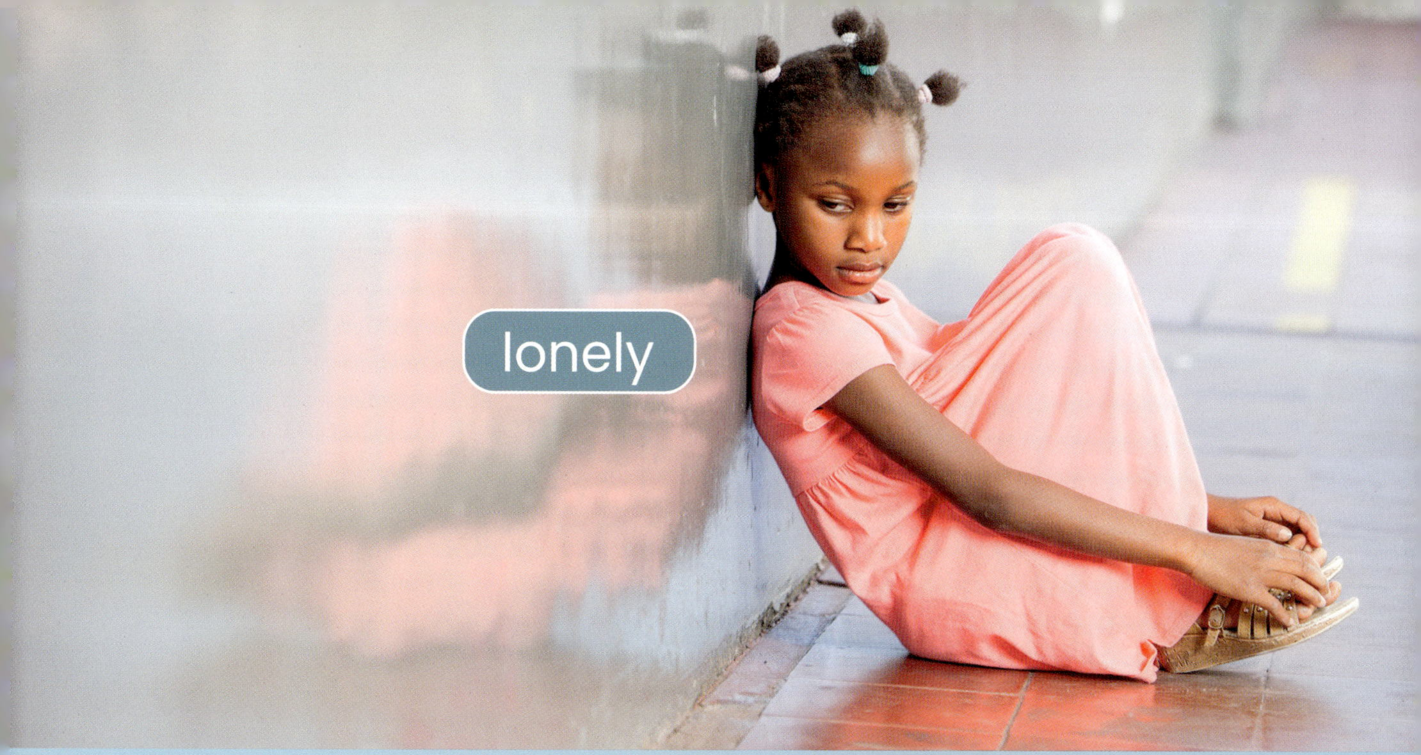
lonely

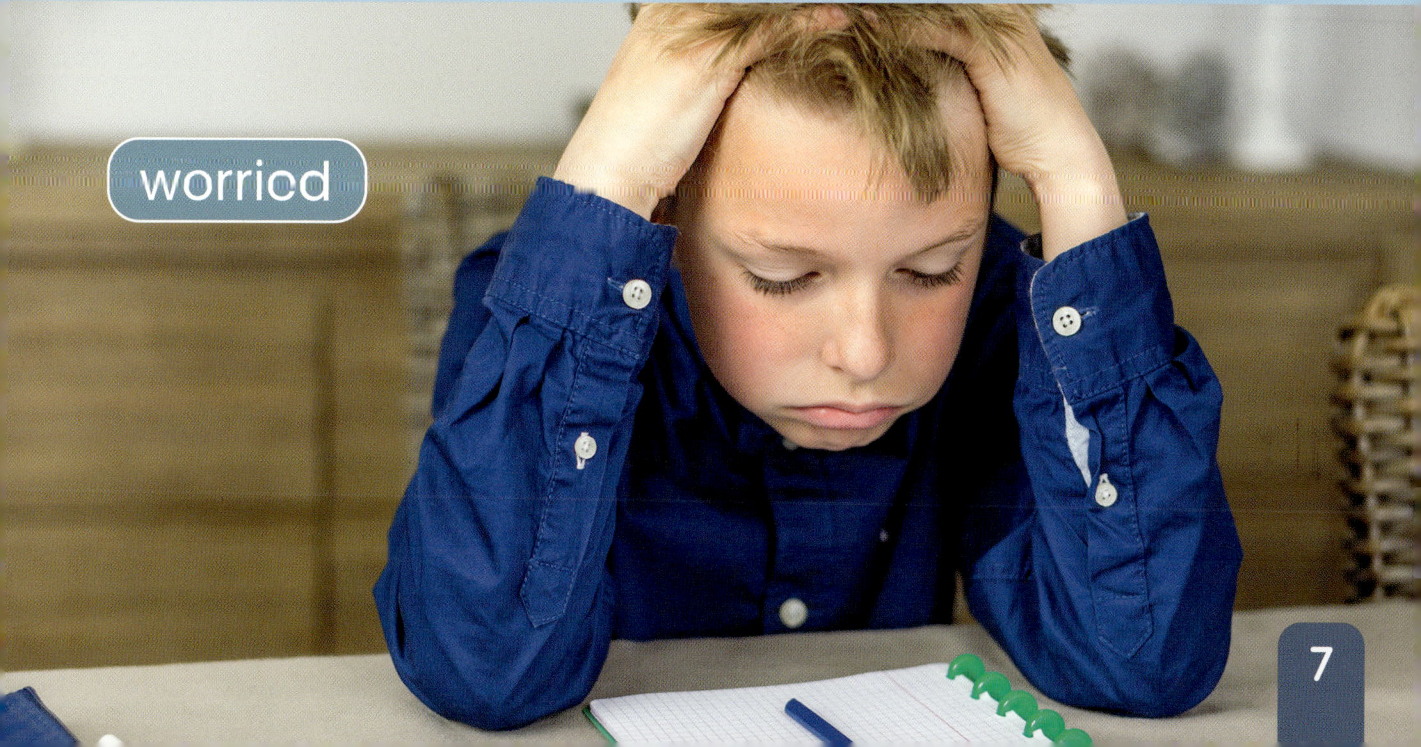
worried

People can learn how to deal with strong feelings. They can learn how to handle hard times. Certain skills are important for mental health. People can practice these skills.

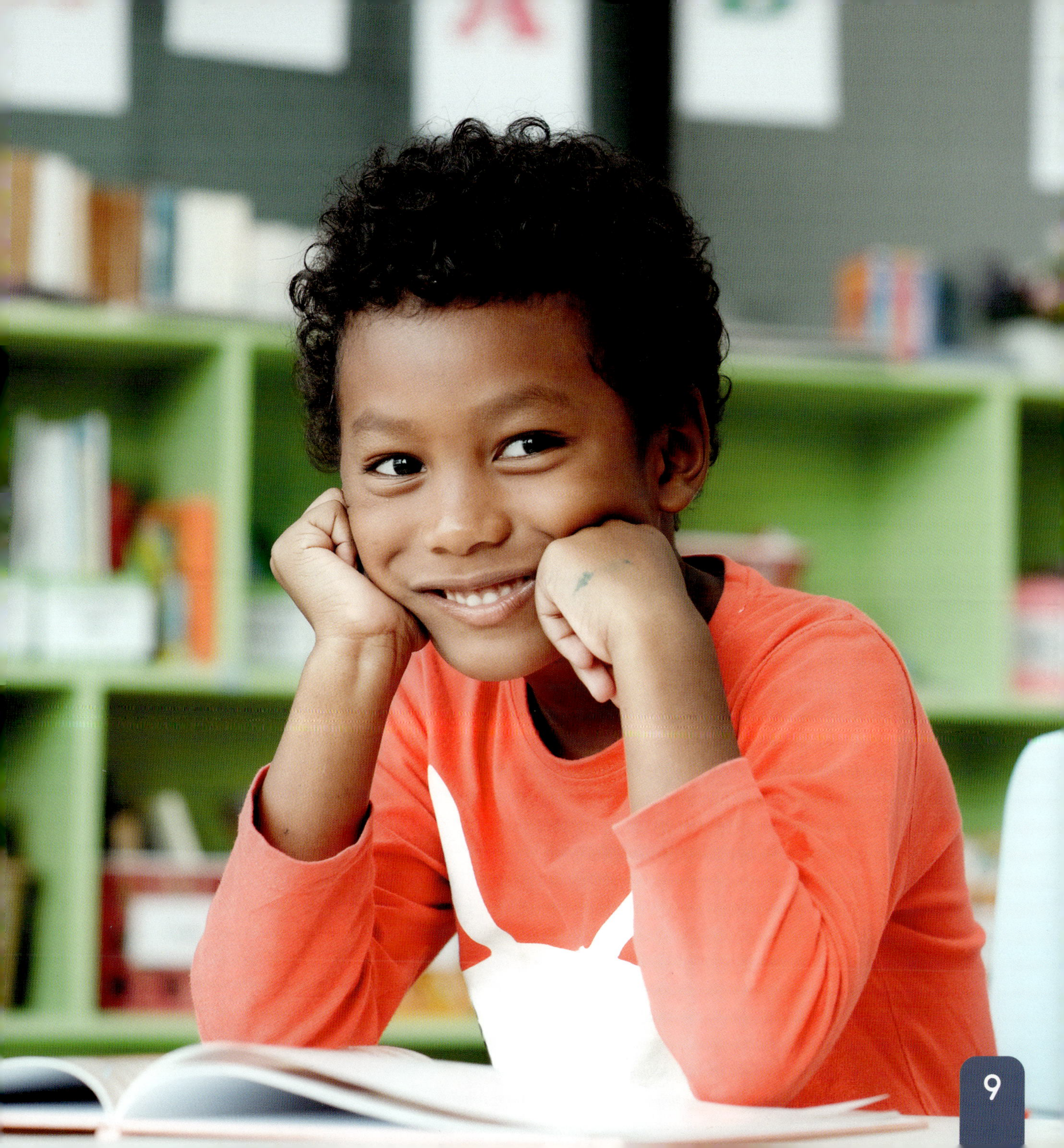

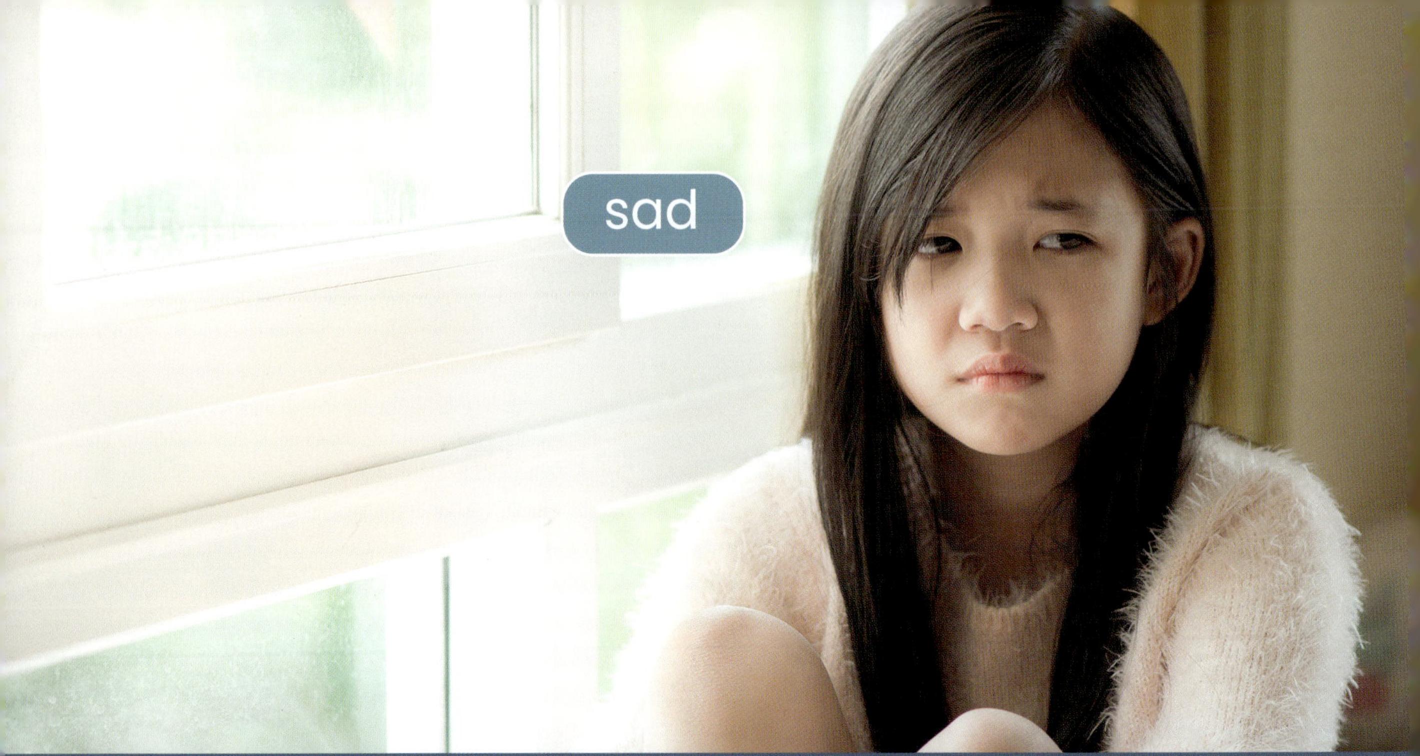
sad

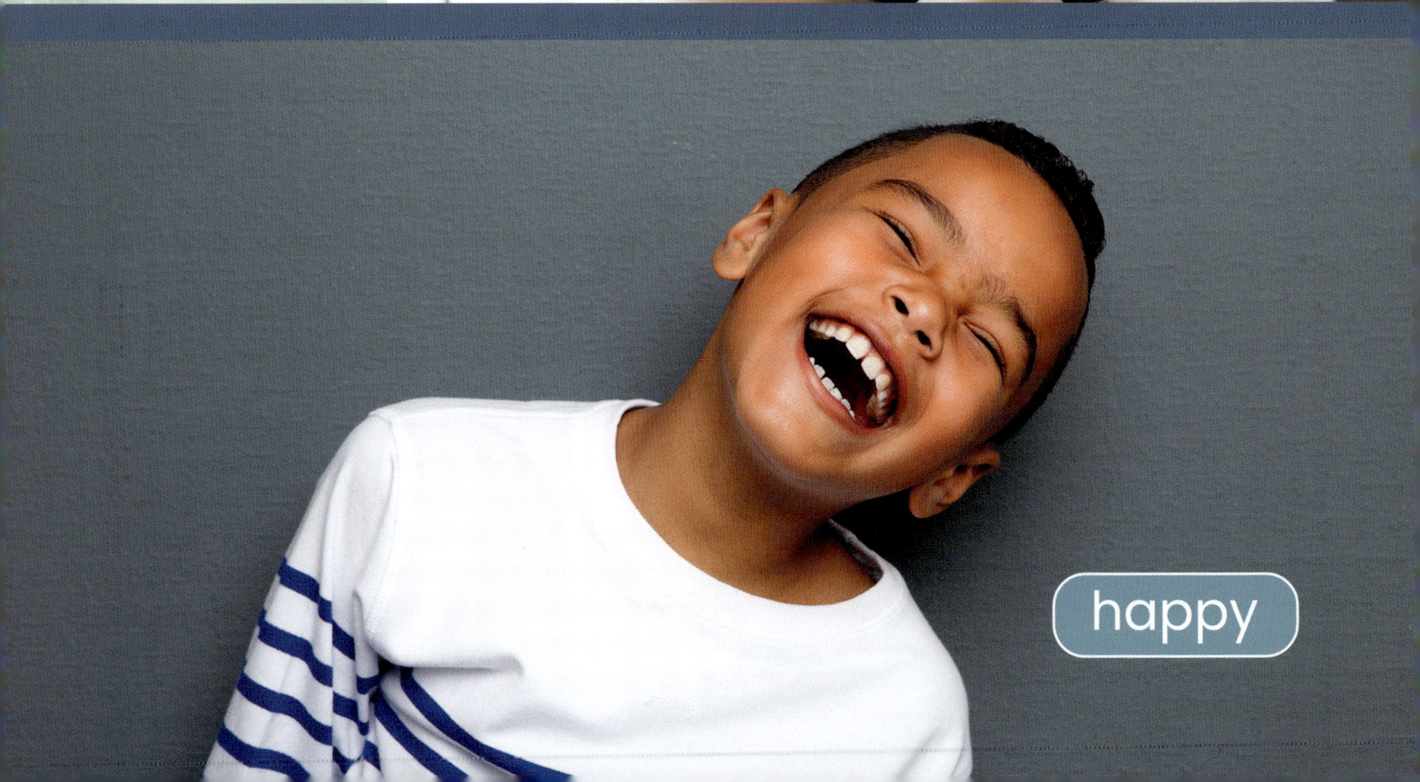
happy

# Name It

One skill is being able to name feelings.

Notice how you feel, and give that feeling a name.

Do you feel sad or happy?

Put the feeling into words.

Think of why you might be feeling that way.
Then share how you feel.
You could say, “I feel sad because my friend can’t play today.”
Or, “I feel happy because we are going to the playground.”

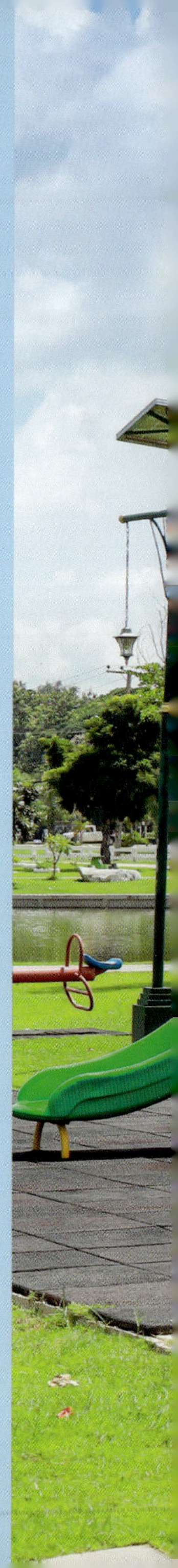

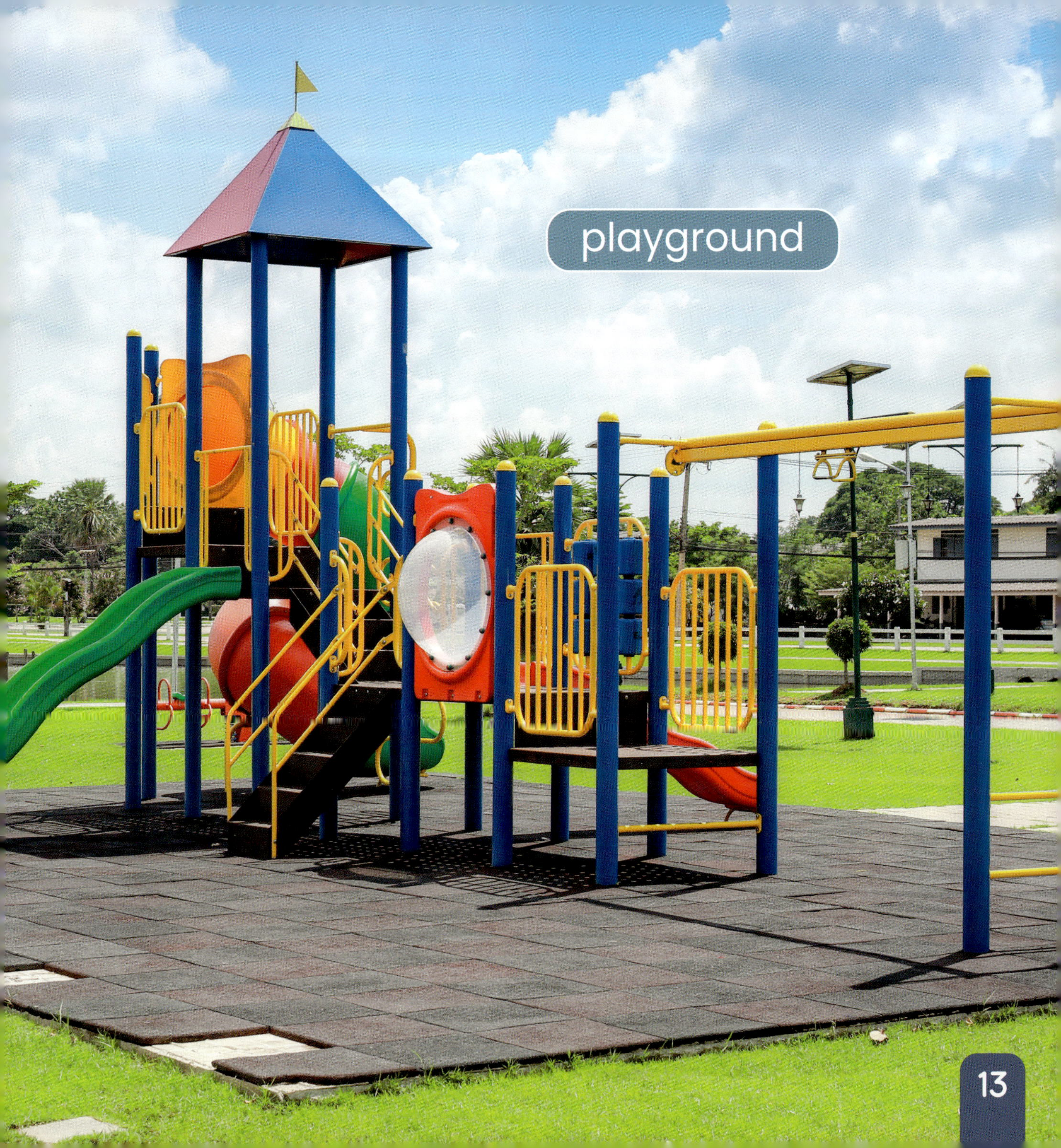
playground

Talking about feelings is an important skill.
It helps people feel close to one another.
Maybe you don’t know how you feel.
That is okay, too.

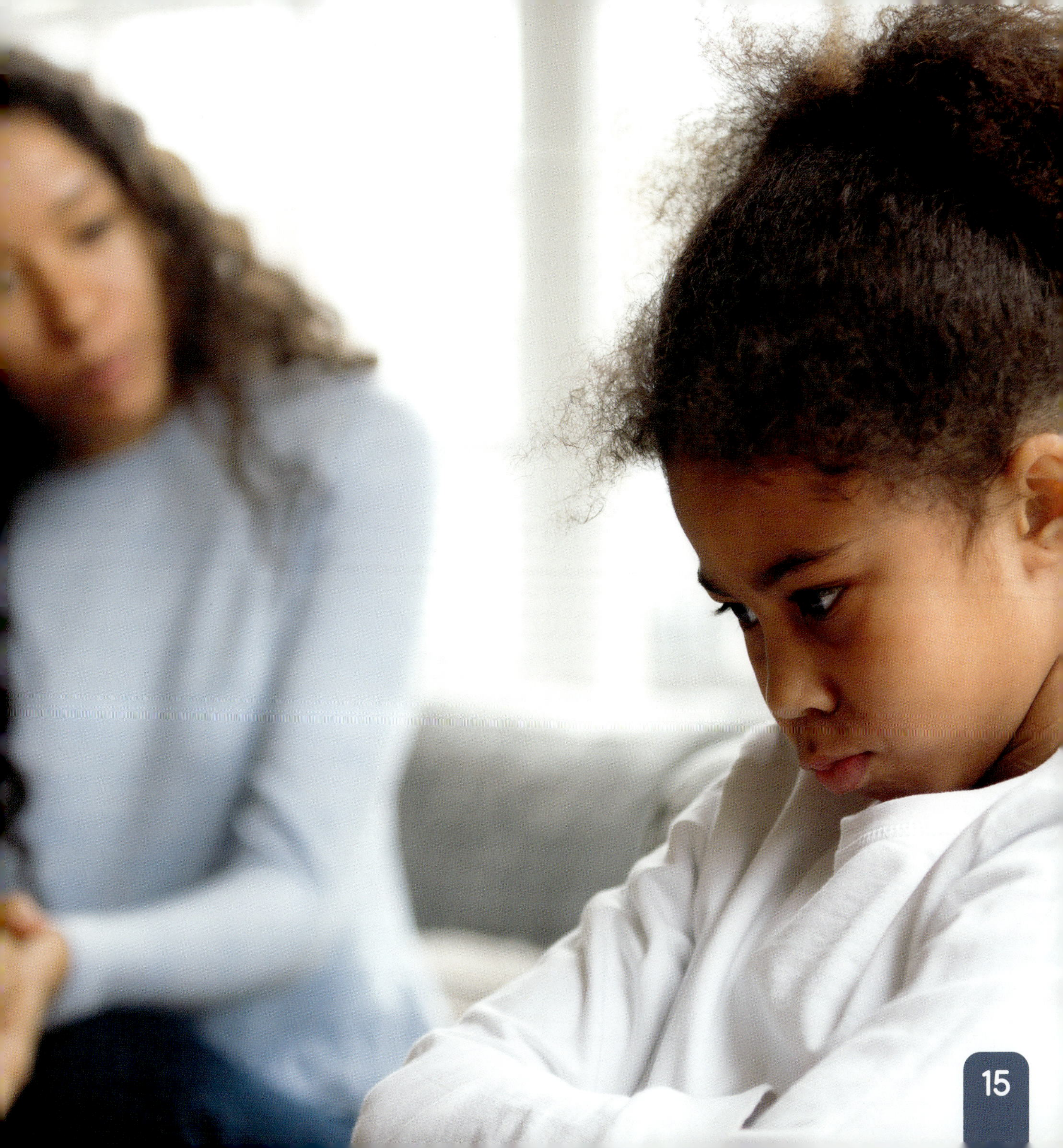

You can still talk with loved ones.
Ask friends or family to listen as you share.
They might be able to help you.
Together, you can figure out what's going on.

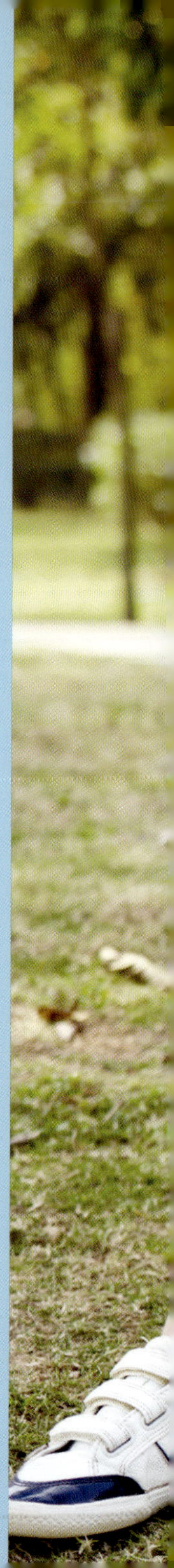

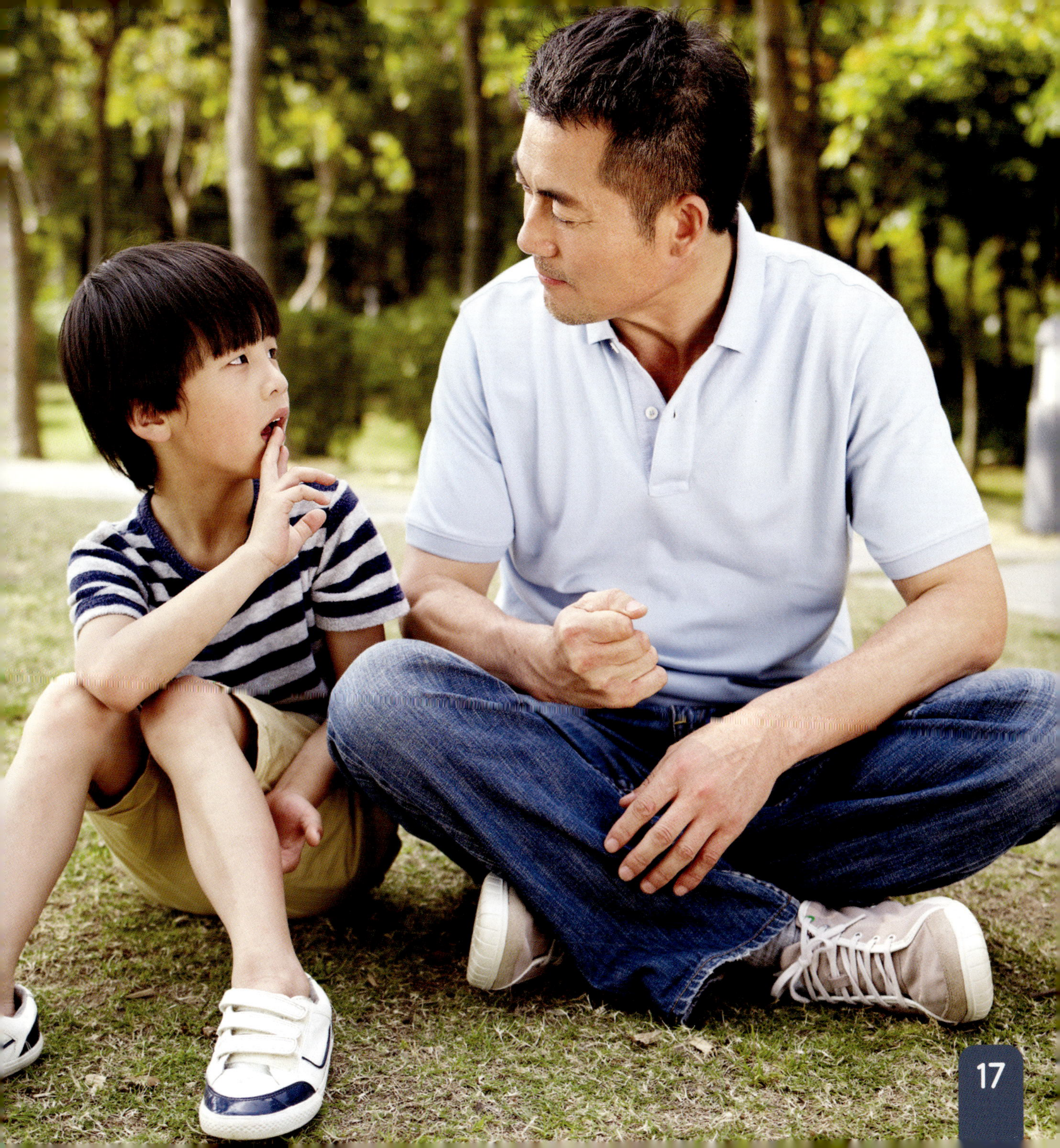

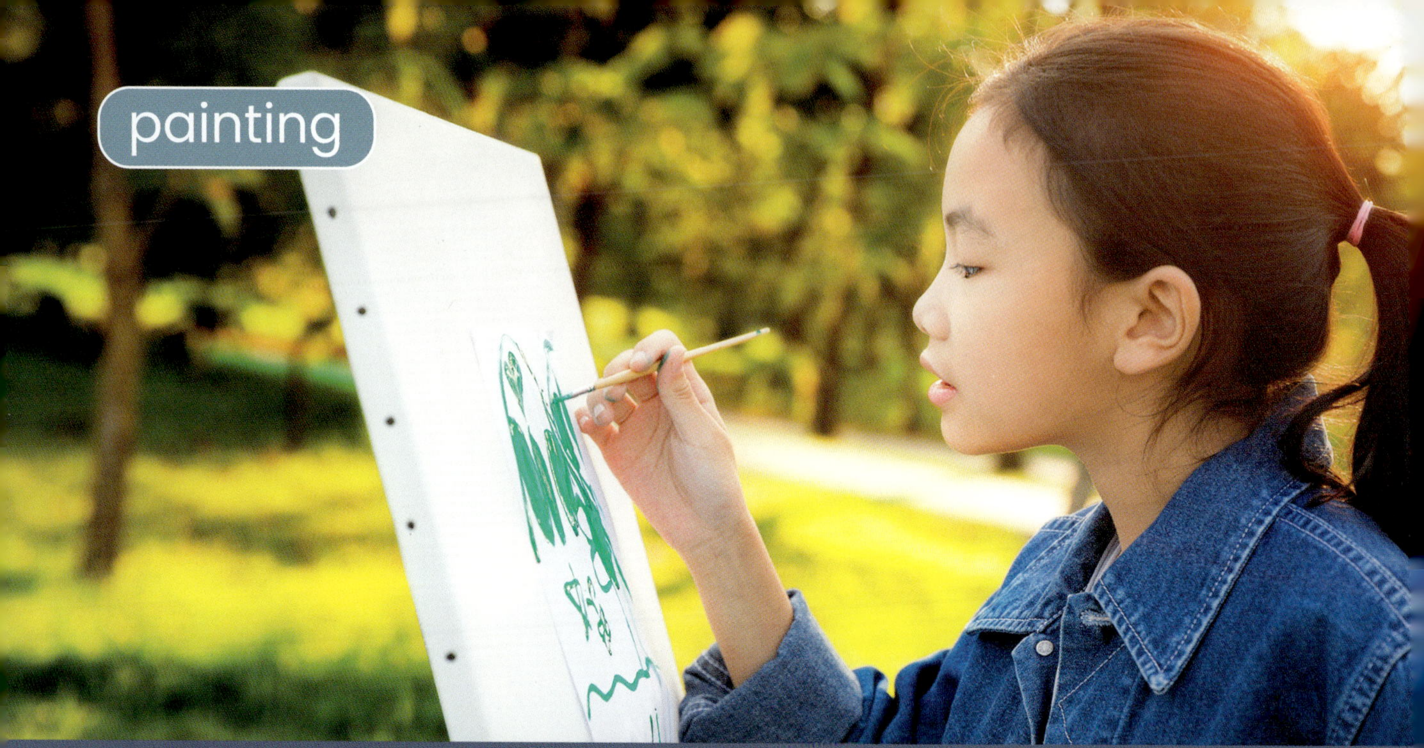
painting

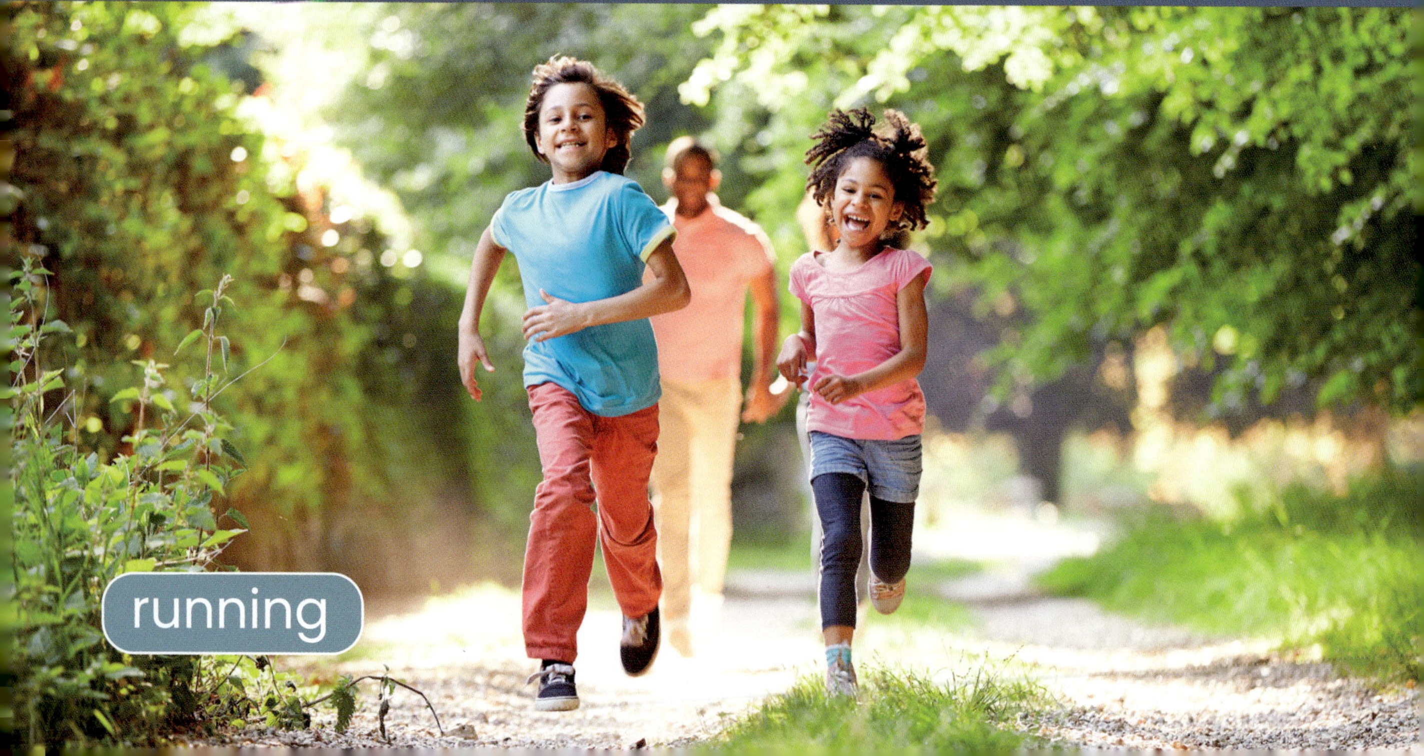
running

# Feel It

Do not try to stop the feeling or hold it inside.

Instead, let the feeling out.

You could paint a picture.

You could run hard to use up energy.

Maybe your feelings are hard to handle.
If so, breathe deeply and count to ten.
Ask a loved one for help.
People care about you, and you are not alone.

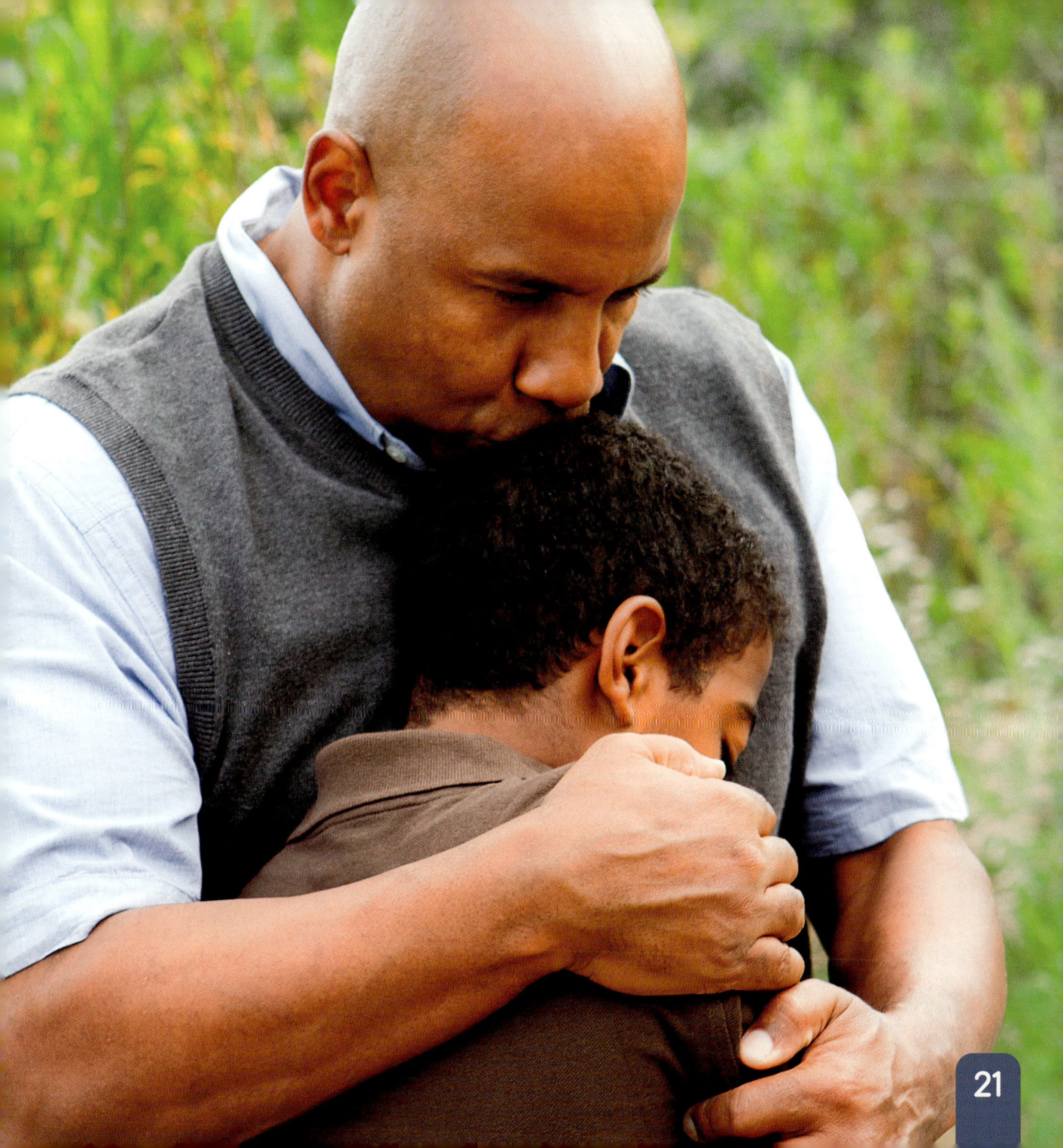

Feelings change often. You might feel one way now. You might feel a different way tomorrow. Practicing mental health will help you live with these feelings.

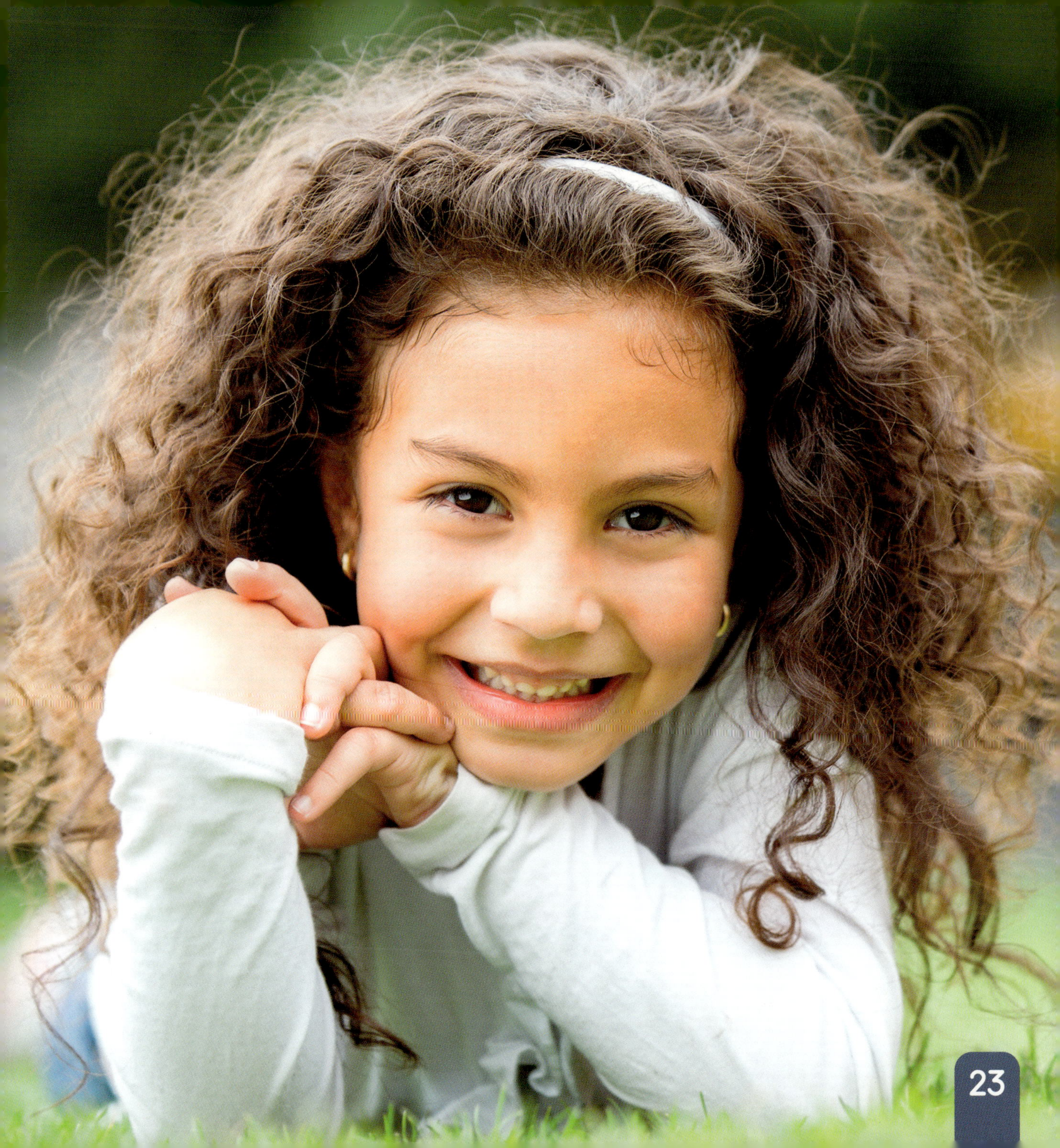

# Glossary

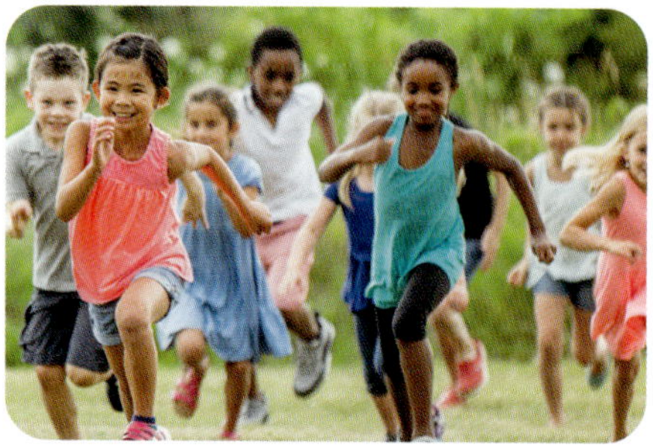

**exercise**

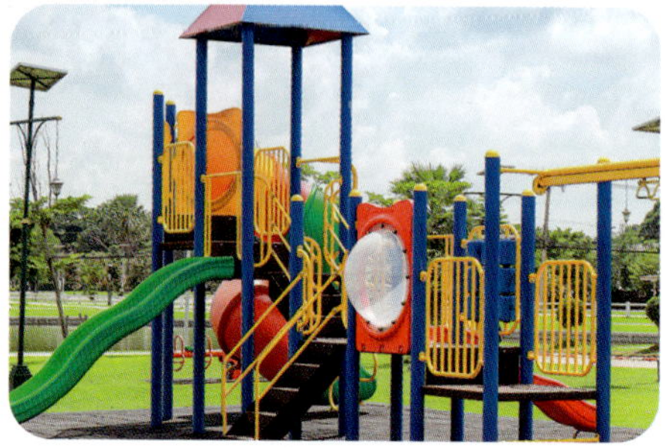

**playground**

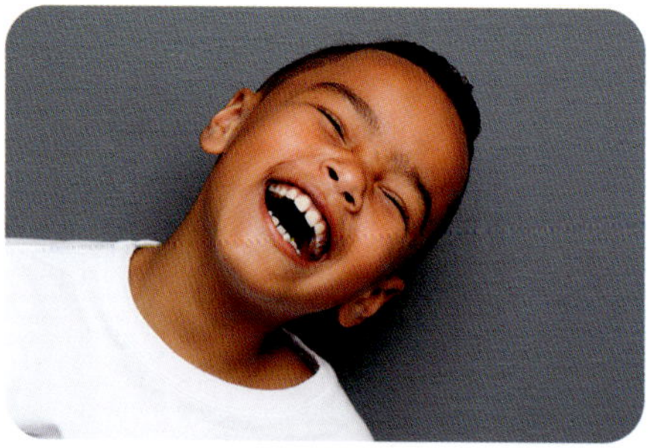

**happy**

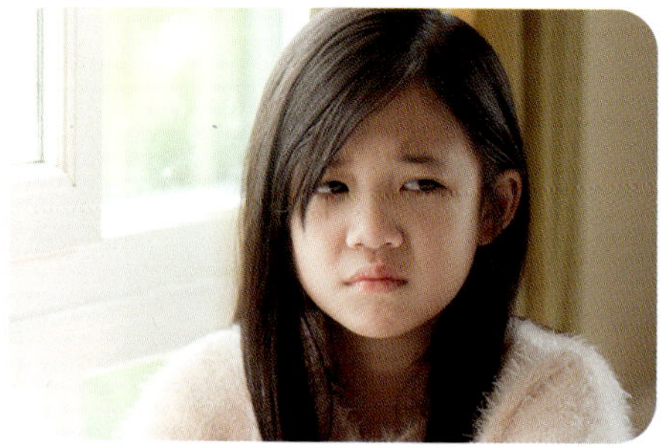

**sad**

# Index